MY NEW FAMILY DOCTOR

THE

URGENT AID CLINIC!

Digital Version Available

ISBN# 1451561989 paperback

# TABLE OF CONTENTS

Dedicated to Jim, Mickey and Victoria

## NOTE TO THE READER

This book is not written for replacement of any medical advises or medical treatment. The reader is advised to consult your own family doctor, or health care professional prior to using any other these suggestions therein. The case study if any are general, the reader must understand that we are all different. We all have different needed and may respond differently to treatment. It's the reader's reasonability to research any and all information.

The format of this book is not in a traditional layout. Each topic has its own header for easy reference. Drop caps are used at the start of each of the chapter's .Text is written in common everyday language so that most readers can read and understand each of the topics. Each topic is a addressed in a short straight to the point manor.

It is recommended that everyone attend a first aid class. This will give you the reader a better understanding of when a medical condition or illness is truly life threatening and urgent. Classes are free in some area of the United States or for a small fee. Check with your local library, and

/or local community center. The internet is also another great tool, classes are now offered online, for a small fee.

## ABOUT THE AUTHOR

M r. Wildfire has a vast understand of our healthcare system spending over twenty years committed to others in need. Viewing patient care at all levels of our health care system. Including major sporting events, concerts, fire departments, ambulance services, clinics and hospitals.

He brings his vast knowledge together to review our current tend in the American health care system. What will soon be our new family doctor the Urgent aid clinics.

# INTRODUCTION

Very few people know where the urgent aid concept came from or was born. All across America urgent aid clinics have popped up. There in shopping malls, on our local street corners and inside our local big box retail stores. The corner clinic offers everything from pre- employment physical, immunization, and fixing broken bones.

In the past 20 years they have grown and become part of your local landscape. Few people have an understanding of how they work, what they can do, or understand their limitations.

The advertizing and marketing boost many different claims. The most common of these is the little or no wait concept, comparing themselves to the local hospitals. Followed by the no appointment needed, compared to your family doctor or most other non urgent aid style clinics like the local county health department. The lower cost option than the local hospital, is the last of the common claims.

As growth and demand continues throughout the United Stated. Each clinic will offer different incentive to visit their clinic instead of their competitors.

We will take a look inside these so called fast urgent aid clinics. Each year hundreds if not thousand of people flock to these urgent aid clinic for some very common and some not so common illness and accidents. In the forgoing chapters we will look at some of these common illness and accidents.

We will offer the reader some tips and pointers on what every consumer should know before walking thru the door of these urgent aid clinics.

## BIRTH THE START OF IT ALL

The urgent aid clinic is new to the everyday consumer. The concept started long ago, in a hospital. When a team of doctors, and hospital directors sat down in a room and reviewed a summary report on the type of customer services it was providing and how long it took to provide those services.  What the analysis report revealed was, that customer needing minor services such as x-rays etc. were waiting to long. While some were just leaving,  without using any of service's from the hospital.

The directors and doctors didn't like this!  It was loss revenue, for the hospital.

As any business person known's you never want the customer to leave with nothing. So they came up with the idea of what they called the fast track. The concept was simple, the consumer who required little in services, chest x-rays, lab test, simple cuts or broken bones. They were taken to this fast track area of the hospital. Instead of having them, waiting beds in the emergency room for these minor services.

By doing this, it did wonders for the hospitals, it increased their profits. It reduced the work load for their staff members. It decreased the waiting time for consumer waiting for services. This made everyone happy.

Soon this concept moved to a free standing building on the hospital grounds. This was the first urgent aid clinic.

The urgent aid clinics offer the consumer a wide verity of services. Each comes with some sort limitations.

As the reader moves a long thru this book we will look at when you should be seen by your family doctor. When you may want to go to the urgent aid clinic or when you should go directly to the hospital, or use emergency services such as 911,

## MARKETING

With approximately 8,725 urgent aid clinic in the United State with a growth rate of about 1,000 new clinics per year. (Keeping in mind there only about 4,500 emergency rooms in the United States)

Millions of dollars are spent each and every year on research of the consumer and likes and dislikes. The urgent aid clinic is not an exception to this. Spending hundreds of thousand of dollars on researching to, find right location for each clinic, and what services are needed for the local area.

The global internet has also helped these clinics grow like wildfire. Their websites offer everything from online registration, online interview, discount offers, free medications, and online timers so you can see what your wait time will be prior to your visit, to the urgent aid clinic, discount coupons, discount memberships, and waiting room by pass. Ask a doctor a question, medical information and treatment. Some of these websites even offer first aid information.

The days of adverting promotional gift items are all most over. The promotional calendars, refrigerator magnets, band aid holders, and logo bags have been replaced by email ads, and road side signs and banners. Some of the larger urgent aid clinics have even used radio and TV ads... The old days of referrals by word of month is rarely used.

Waiting room bypass is a very different approach to the standard clinic waiting room wait. By completing your information online, you will then be asked when would like to schedule your appointment. Since you have taken the time to pre-register you can pick your time and bypass anyone who is in the waiting room already.

Sounds like a great idea but, since this is a new concept a not well known or widely used. It will be a wait and see game, as to how will impact the clinic performance time..

As the ownership grows in these franchises, so will all the target marketing. Owners will try different marketing approaches to keep old consumers and attract new ones.

# WEBSITES

With the global internet at the consumers finger tips, this has provided the consumer a wealth of information.

Each of the urgent aid clinics website offers different information, services, and facts. Very few of urgent aid clinics owners own just one clinic. Your local urgent aid clinic may offer one or more of the following services or information on the clinic's website.

About Us
Ask a Question.
Authorization
Frequently Asked Questions
Fee Schedule
Find a Doctor
Free stuff
HIPAA Notice
History
Hours of Operation
Insurance
Career Openings
Corporate Care
Discount Coupons
Maps and Locations
Meet the Staff

News alerts
Pay My Bill
Pre-Register
Request an estimate

The list will be endless, as new online services and information are added each and every day. Check out all the websites for urgent aid clinic in your area. You may find that one provider offers more of the services you need then it competitors offer. You also may find a better price for the same services.

## OWNERSHIP

Most everyone would like to think that the urgent aid clinic that they are visiting is owned by a healthcare professional. But this may not be the case.

Very few states require that an urgent aid clinic actually be owned by a licensed Physician.

Other states allow corporation to own a clinics as long as the corporation employs medical professionals in the clinic as required by that state standards of care.

Some states have passed strict laws on how urgent aid clinic can market their clinic to the general public. Today most of the urgent aid clinic ownership is made up of, Physicians, Hospitals and Corporations or a combination of any of these.

As the current trend of easy access to health care becomes more profitable, you will find that more and more of the clinics will be owned by groups of business persons or corporate share holders instead of health care professionals.

# WALK –IN

Let start our review as most people do with a walk into the urgent aid clinic. Depending on your local community you may find a large or small waiting area.

It will look like most other doctor's offices, rows of chairs and an endless stack of magazines. Some have televisions so you can catch up on your missed television shows. Some clinics even run their own info commercial in their waiting rooms.

When you walk up to the front desk a receptionist is the first people you will meet in the clinic. The receptionist will greet you and ask for identification, insurance information and the reason for your visit.

You will be asked if you have ever been in the clinic before. If you're new you may be asked to fill out a detailed history. Urgent aid clinic are getting away from having the consumer fill out a history form.

Returning clients may or may not have there old chart records pulled for viewing by the health care provider. In our computer age, very few clinics use paper hand written charting anymore.

In some area of the country you can pre-register online and fill out information in advance for your visit to the urgent aid clinic. Some urgent aid clinics allow you to update your personal information, as well as your medical information.

After the receptionist verifies your insurance is active, you will be asked to pay any co-pays required by your health insurance plan. If you have any outstanding balance you will need to settle this as well. After all this has been completed you will then be seen by a health care provider.

# THE INTERVIEW

You will be called back into and exam room by one of the clinic staff members. The clinic staff is a generic term used to describe a wide verity a member staff members that work in the clinics. Each of the staff members that you may come in contact with is covered in greater detail in the section called clinical staff.

The clinic staff starts with a review of any medical information that you filed out, prior to bring you back into the exam room. The interview is where you will state the reason for your visit. The clinic staff member will ask additional questions about your condition. This interview information is what the provider will review prior to treating you. You must be clear, honest, and detailed. During the interview process your blood pressure may be checked as well as your pulse. Some clinics may require a eye exam and check your height and weight. The clinic staff will asked you about any surgery you may have had, your medical history, medication you are current taking, any allergy's you have, and your family medical history etc.

# MEDICAL HISTORY

Your medical history tells the story for your body. You're the best person to ask when it comes to this. It will help the provider understand your body and how it responds to medical treatments.

It is important to keep current and accurate medical history on yourself and your family. Your medical history should include medications, surgeries, allergies to medications and any medical condition you are being treated for or have been treated for in the past...

Everyone should bring this list with them each and every visit. to the any clinic, urgent aid clinic, doctor's office, or hospital.

All this information can be put on an index card and stored in your wallet or purse.

At the end of this book, a check list has been provided for you to build your own medical history information sheet.

Some people feel that since the urgent aid clinic is not their family doctor they don't need to tell them everything. about their history, medications or any past treatments.

Withholding information can affect proper treatment of your condition. You should always provide a full medical history whenever you visit any health care professional for any treatments.

# MEDICATION

Most people are very good when it comes to remember things. But sometimes our mind forgets things.  Keep a list of your medications as well was your families with you at all times. This list should include of any medication you are taking including any over the counter medications if you're in a hurry for time, just bring the medication bottles with you to the clinic If you have children make a list for them.

This list should include the full name of the medication, the strength and how often you are required to take the medication, and why you're taking the medication.

Medication can do many different things, cure infections, stop pain and discomfort. But too many medications can cause serious health problem.

Your family doctor has a list of all your medications and has been treating you and your family for a long time.  You should consult your family doctor before starting any new medication or treatment, or any changes in your current medication treatment.

Over medication often comes from treatment for a condition when the consumer is seen by many different doctors. You should avoid this! Get in the habit of asking the doctor what this medication will do, and why you are taking this medication.

People have sometimes put a blind trust in doctors. Here is an example a older lady come into the clinic for treatment. When asked what the medications she was taking, she pulled out a pill box labeled for everyday of the week. She proceed to say that she takes two red ones, one green one each morning then in the evening she takes one yellow, one red and one of the green pills.. When she was asked what are these medications for? She said "I don't know the doctor told me to take them."

## FAMILY HISTORY

Your family history may seem unimportant to you when you are being seen at an urgent aid clinic. But your family's history provides the health care provider with insight to possible additional causes to your current condition or illness..

For example frequent urination may mean a urinary track infection, but if you have a family history of diabetes, this may also indicate the start of new diabetic condition.

Please use the guild lines outlined at the end of this book to make your own family history list.

# ALLERGIES

Allergy is an immune system disorder. Reaction can range from mild to severe life threatening and potentially to death.

Treatment should start by avoiding the allergen in question or reducing exposure to it. Symptoms can sometimes be managed and treated with over the counter medication. Severe reaction such as shortness of breath, hives should seek immediate medical attention preferably a hospital emergency room, or call emergency services (911) for help.

Learning and tracking of all your allergies will help prevent any complications to any condition you may have. When you visit the urgent aid clinic or seek medical attention for any illness or injury, if the clinical staff doesn't ask you what your allergies are, make sure you tell them.

Now that you have given the clinical staff all your information, the first part has finished. You will now wait in the room until the provider comes in.

The provider will review your information that you gave to the clinic staff prior to meeting with you. The provider will again review your information with you. The provider may take a look in your ears, and mouth, listening to your heart etc.

After reviewing any findings of the exam with you the provider may, request additional testing. If not, the provider will advise you of a treatment plan. This may include medication for the treatment of your condition or illness.

## PROVIDER

The provider is a blanket term used to describe the PA, MD, or DO.

Sometimes people feel uneasy in explaining their medical condition or illness during the internal interview with the clinic staff.

Keep in mind that omissions can affect the treatment plan you receive. After the provider has finished the exam is the wrong time to bring up additional information.

## EXIT INTERVIEW

Your exit interview is where a clinic staff member will review your discharge instructions with you. This may include a treatment plan for you to follow at home.

When the clinical staff member will returns with your discharge instruction and any prescriptions for you. This is your last chance to ask any question about your treatment plan, so please make sure you understand everything before the clinic staff leaves.

You are now done so you walk out the clinic and get back in your car. Hopefully all in under an hour or two..

# CLINICAL STAFF

The clinic staff you meet during your visit may have a wide verity of medical training. They may include CNA, and MA. EMT, PARAMEDIC, RN, NP, PAC, MD, and DO we will take a look at each of these clinic staff members as we move along.

Keep in mind each of the 50 states have different regulation and requirements for each of the clinic staff member.

## CERTIFIED NURSING ASSISTANT (CNA)

The Nursing Assistant is an important member of the clinic's health care staff who often holds a high level of experience and ability. Common basic tasks may include any of the following. Vital signs, provide patient care by applying dressings. Prepare patients for, treatment, or examination.

# MEDICAL ASSISTANT (MA)

Medical assistants are not licensed professionals they are required to work under the direct supervision of a licensed physician, registered nurse, nurse practitioner or physician assistant whenever they provide direct (hands-on) patient care procedures.

Medical assistants perform many administrative duties, including, greeting patients, filing patients' medical records,, scheduling appointments, laboratory services,. Duties vary according to state law and may include taking medical histories and recording vital signs, explaining treatment to patients, preparing patients for examination, and assisting during diagnostic examinations.

Medical assistants may collect and prepare laboratory specimens or perform basic laboratory test..They instruct patients about medications, prepare and administer medications as directed, authorize drug refills as directed, telephone prescriptions to a pharmacy, draw blood, prepare patients for X-rays, take electrocardiograms, and change dressings.

## EMT-B (basic)

EMT-Basic is the entry level of EMS The procedures and skills allowed at this level are generally non-invasive such as bleeding control, supplemental oxygen administration, and splinting  Some medications, training requirements and treatment protocols vary from area to area, and state to state.

## EMT-I (Intermediate)

EMT-Intermediates .training allows several more invasive procedures including IV therapy, the use of multi-lumen airway devices and provides for enhanced assessment skills.

## EMT-P (Paramedic)

Paramedic represents the highest level of EMT, and in general, the highest level of pre-hospital medical provider. Paramedics perform a variety of medical procedures such as fluid resuscitation, pharmaceutical administration, obtaining IV access, cardiac monitoring and other advanced procedures and assessments

# REGISTERD NURSE (RN)

The scope of practice of a registered nurses is determined by Nurse Practice Act. Each state has its own laws, rules, and regulations governing nursing care. It should be noted that in some states the terms "nurse" or "nursing" may only be used in conjunction with the practice of a Registered Nurse (RN) or licensed practical or vocational nurse (LPN/LVN).

## NURSE PRACTITIONERS (NP)

Nurse Practitioner (NP) is a registered nurse who has completed specific advanced nursing education (master's degree) and training in the diagnosis and management of common as well as a few complex medical conditions.

## PHYICIAN ASSISTANT (PAC)

Is a healthcare professional licensed to practice medicine with supervision of a licensed physician. Physician assistants have their own medical licenses and do not work under a physician's license. Physician supervision can be direct, or by phone, or any other reliable means. The physician supervision, in most cases, need not be direct or on-site. Many PAs practice in remote or underserved areas in satellite clinics.

## DOCTOR OF MEDICINE (MD)

This is your family; a Doctor of Medicine is a four-year graduate-level academic degree for physicians and surgeons in the United States.

## DOCTOR OF OSTEOPATHIC MEDICINE (DO)

Doctor of Osteopathic Medicine, are trained much in the same way as M.D.'s, with the addition of <u>osteopathic manipulative medicine</u> techniques.

## X-RAY TECH

Radiologic technicians perform imaging examinations like X rays while technologists use other imaging modalities such as computed tomography, magnetic resonance imaging, and mammography.

## LICENSE TO PRACTICE MEDICINE

The above heading says it all, keep this in mind when you visit any health care clinic or hospital. Your doctor has a license to practice some times they make error as we all do from time to time.

You should consider a second option or consult your family doctor if there has been no improvement in your condition from any medical treatment.

# INSURANCE

Most urgent aid clinic will accept most medical insurance plans, Medicare and Medicaid are sometimes accepted. For those without insurance you will be asked to pay cash for any services provided.

If you're insurance plan requires any co-pay this will be collected before you are seen by the clinic staff.

We will take a fast look at the types of insurance plan on the market today. You should take the time to understand your insurance plan, for each policy or plan has different restrictions and limitations. Finding out at the last minute what is not covered, can set you up for some major financial problems.

Note to the reader this book was written prior to the health reform act passes in 2010.

## FEE FOR SERVICE

This is the traditional kind of health care plan. Where the insurance company pay's for the services provided. A deductible must be paid before the insurance company payments will begin. The deductible might be as little as $250 or as high as $1,000 for each member of your family.

After you have paid your deductible, you will then share part the bill with the insurance company. For example, you might pay 30 % while the insurance company pays 70 %. Some services maybe limited or not covered at all.

It is a good idea to check your coverage prior to your visit to a clinic or hospital. This may prevent some unneeded financial expense.

# HMO's

Health maintenance organizations are prepaid health plans. As an HMO member, you pay a monthly premium.

The HMO arranges for care either directly in its own group practice and/or through doctors and other health care professionals under contract.

There may be a small co-payment for each office visit, such as $5 for a doctor's visit or $25 for hospital emergency room treatment.

Because HMOs receive a fixed fee for your covered medical care, it is in their interest to make sure you get basic health care for problems before they become serious.

Keep in mind that you are pre paying to be seen by your family doctor! If are seen by any other doctor your insurance company may not pay for any part of your bill.

## PREFERRED PROVIDER ORGANIZATION (PPOs)

The preferred provider organization is a combination of traditional fee-for-service and an HMO. When you use their providers, most of your medical bills are covered.

Some insurance company will not pay any insurance claim if you go outside their doctor network.

# MEDICARE

The Medicare program was developed by the government to help those who are eligible with their overwhelming health care bills.

It is funded by every tax payer as part of your payroll taxes.

## THE ORIGINAL MEDICARE PLAN

The federal government manages the Original Medicare Plan. It operates on a fee-for-service plan. Most people pay a deductible and then a co-pay or co-insurance. Medicare offer different plans each cover different things, but all may have a monthly fee or deductible. This may include Medicare Advantage Plan Medicare Advantage Plan or Plan C combines your Part A and B coverage, but is provided by private insurance companies.

## Part A

Part A is hospital insurance provided by Medicare. Covers most of the patient care in nursing home's, ,hospital's, hospice and home health care.

## Part B

Part B is medical insurance to pay for medically necessary services and supplies provided by Medicare. Most people will have to pay a premium to receive this coverage. Part B covers outpatient care, doctor's services, physical or occupational therapists, and additional home health care.

## Part C

Part C is the combination of Part A and Part B. The main difference in Part C is that it is provided through private insurance companies approved by Medicare.

## Part D

Part D is stand-alone prescription drug coverage insurance. Most people do have to pay a premium for this coverage.

Original Medicare Plans do not cover everything. Costs that you may incur include co-insurance, co-pays, deductibles, etc. These costs are sometimes called gaps. To help cover these costs you might want to buy a Medicare insurance gap policy.

## MEDICAID

Medicaid health insurance provides health care coverage for some low-income people who cannot afford it. Medicaid sends payments directly to your health care providers.

Medicaid is a Federal program that is operated by the States. Each individual state decides who is eligible and the scope of health services offered.

## INSURANCE CO-PAYS

Almost every insurance company has a co-pay for visit. A co-pay or co-payment is the amount you must pay for your use of a medical service covered by your policy. This can range from $5.00 to $1,500.00 or more.

Most insurance companies have added urgent aid clinic to their list of co-pay services. But keep in mind that if the consumer needs additional services more than what the urgent aid clinic can offer additional co-pay will be required.

## COMMON ILLINESS/INJURY

In the forgoing pages are the most common reasons people have visited the urgent aid clinic. The information herein are suggestions and common sense should be used by the reader.

You should contact your family doctor or any healthcare provider about any condition or question you may have. This book is **_not_** a replacement for medical treatment or advice and should not be used as such..

# ABDOMINAL PAIN

Abdominal pain (or stomach ache) Diagnosis of the cause of abdominal pain can be difficult, because many diseases can result in this symptom of pain. Abdominal pain is a common problem.

Acute abdomen pain can be defined as severe, persistent abdominal pain of sudden onset. The pain may also include nausea and vomiting, abdominal distention, fever and signs of shock. One of the most common conditions associated with acute abdominal pain is acute appendicitis.

A medical evaluation will be needed by a health care provider.

# ACNE

Is a common skin condition affecting the face, chest, arms and even the back. The condition is caused by oil glands in the skin that become plugged. A common myth is that acne is caused by food, but some foods can make it worse.

Good hygiene is the best preventive measure. Wash the affected area with unscented soap at least three times a day.

Shampoo your hair at least four times a week. After exercising or any heavy work, shower to wash off any sweats and oils. Avoid cosmetics, if possible use water based if any.

Don't squeeze, scratch or pick at the skin. Over the counter treatment can help control mild acne.

Severe acne or where over the counter treatment has failed a dermatologist is recommended. Treatments both over the counter or prescribed may take 4 to 6 weeks before any results are seen

# ABCESS

This is an infection under your skin. This can be treated by medication or removing the fluid from the area as well. Sometimes both treatments are needed. This can be take one visit or can require multiple return visits.

# BIRTH CONTROL

Some states allow providers to provide or prescribe these medications. Most all require a parents consent if the consumer is under 18. Contact your local health department for information in your area of the country.

# BITES

Animal or human bites can happen anywhere. There maybe breaks and punctures in the skin with deep cut or bruises. Small bites with controlled bleeding can be well taken care of at the urgent aid clinics. Larger, multiple, bites or uncontrolled should be treat at the hospital or contact emergency services.

## BLADDER INFECTION (UTI)

Bladder infection is an infection of the urinary tract. Women are more likely to have a bladder infection then men. Symptoms may include increase urination, pain or pressure upon urination, strong odor, lower back pain, chills, fever, and sweat.

Treatment is with antibiotics and pain medication. Symptoms clear up with 2 to 3 days after medication has started.

Contact your family doctor if no improvement within 3 days you're your condition gets worse.

## BONE FRACTURE

Bone fracture is a break in the bone. Signs and symptoms may include one or more of the following, pain, swelling, tenderness, deformity, bleeding, weakness or numbness.

Treatment should include calling 911 for help. Give first aid treatment to control any bleeding. Apply ice to reduce any swelling.

Never try fix or straighten any deformity, or try to set the bone yourself.

Most facture will require casts, splints, or special braces to heal. Hospital treatment will be needed for severe fractures.

## BRONCHITIS

Most bronchitis can be treated with medication therapy. Should shortness of breath occur, hospitalization may be required.

# BURNS

Burns can come from skin contact from chemicals, electricity, heat, radiation, and sunlight.

Minor burn to the skin can be treated at your local urgent aid clinic. Sever burns or burns covering a large amount of the body should be treated at your local hospital or contact emergency services.

For minor burns flush the affected area with cold water for at least 15 minutes. This will reduce pain and swelling. Don't break any blisters! Wrap the area with clean or sterile dressing. Keep the area clean and dry.

# COLDS

Everyone at one time or another has come down with a common cold. Sore throat, sneezing, headache: cough, runny nose, and a fever of less than 100.0.

Cold symptoms develop over a few days. Influenza or the flu have muscle aches also, but these symptoms come on in a few hours not days.

There is no cure for a cold. Antibiotic do not work on a cold. Over the counter medication can be used to treat your symptoms. A cold should run its course in about 1 to 2 weeks. During this time you should get plenty of rest. Drink lots of water, juices etc. (no alcohol)

Call your doctor if any of your symptoms get worse or you develop additional symptoms.

# DIARRHEA

Acute or frequent loose bowel movements start suddenly and stop in a few days. Prolonged diarrhea lasting for than a few day's, may be the sign of other problems. It may also come with a fever or cramps or abdominal pain. Dehydration is can lead to serous problems. Drink plenty of fluids. Contact your family doctor if your symptoms get worse, if you notice blood or if it don't clear up after a few days

Diarrhea is usually controlled by limiting intake to clear fluids only. Avoid all dairy products and citrus fruit juices. Gradually increase the diet as improvement occurs after 24 to 48 hours. Notify your Doctor right away, or go to the Emergency Room in case of the following: Any inability to keep fluids down. Abdominal pain, especially if in the right lower side of the abdomen. Change in mental status, too sleepy, confused, short of breath, more irritable or fussy, slurred speech, and difficulty walking, blood in the stool or vomit.

## EAR INFECTIONS OR PAIN

Ear infections are most common in children and infants. The infection is usually caused by bacteria.

Treatment, not all infections need antibiotic! Medication treatment may be needed, finish all medication prescribed! Even if the symptoms are gone. Most common reason the ear infection returns in a few days or weeks is that the medication was not finished.

## FEVER

Fever can come from many different origin like infection's .Fevers should not necessarily be treated by a health care provider, most people recover without medical attention.

Over the counter medication can be used to reduce the fever. Preventing dehydration during this time you should drink extra fluids while you have the fever.

High fevers of 101 or above which are not controlled by over the counter medications or have lasted 3 or more days you should contact your family doctor.

# HEADACHES

Headaches can be caused by many different things including stress, tension, and infections such as colds. Rarely headaches may be due to bleeding or tumors in the brain.

Headache treatment includes over the counter medicines for pain. Rest, cold or hot packs on painful areas of the head and neck, and massage of the sore muscles may help.

If you have a fever, chills, repeated vomiting, difficulty with vision, unusual numbness or weakness severe pain despite medicine. You should call your family doctor.

# HEARTBURN

Heartburn is the sensation of food coming back up in the throat. It can include belching acid taste in the mouth. Often it's with a heavy burning feeling in the chest. Heartburn can begin within a few hours after eating and may last for hours. Over the counter medication can reduce the discomfort and symptoms.

Heartburn may need to be treated by your family doctor with stronger medication, additional test may rule out conditions known as GERD. Your family doctor may also suggest life style changes needed to reduce your symptoms

# HEAT STROKE

Heatstroke is true emergency! Calling 911 will give the immediate help needed, and provide transportation to the nearest hospital.

Heatstroke is your body is unable to cool itself down anymore. Skin is hot, dry, and flush. There is no sweating, a high body temperature, with a rapid heart beat, confusion may follow or loss consciousness. Dizziness, tiredness, headaches may have all preceded this event.

Rapid cooling of the body is needed, and IV fluids. Do not force anything by mouth. Give cool water, only if the person can drink it themselves.

# HEMORRHIODS

Hemorrhoids are swollen veins in the rectal area that sometimes bleed. Although the cause of hemorrhoids is not always known, it usually comes with constipation and straining to have a bowel movement.

Uncomplicated hemorrhoids are painless but sometimes cause bright red rectal bleeding with a bowel movement. Bleeding is usually a small amount of blood.

Hot baths for at least 15 minutes three times per day and after each bowel movement are the best way to relieve pain and swelling. Use of topical antibiotics, anesthetics or steroidal creams is of limited value.

ncrease fluids and fiber in your diet to keep your bowel movements regular and soft. Use stool softeners and avoid straining on the toilet.

Contact your family doctor if pain increase, hard lumps develops, rectal bleeding is heavy.

# HERPES ZOSTER

Herpes zoster is a condition that causes pain, rash or blistering on the skin. Rash can appear on the chest, arms and legs.

Shingles as it is commonly known happens only in people who have had the chickenpox.

The rash clears up in about 21 days. Nerve pain can last for months. Over the counter treatment can reduce the itching and pain. Additional medical treatment may be needed for increase pain and itching.

# INFLUENZA

Influenza or flu is a viral infection affecting nose, throat, and lungs. Flu symptoms are more severe and can cause severe medical problems.

Influenza symptoms start suddenly. With chills and fever (101.0 or higher) sweating muscle aches may include: runny nose, congestion, cough and a sore throat.

Influenza can usually be diagnosed based on your symptoms. Very few health care providers will use lab test or onsite testing. Most find these tests costly and unnecessary

Most symptoms can be managed at home. It is a good idea to speak to your family doctor if you have symptoms of the flu.

Some providers feel that because fever is part of the immune system's reaction to infection, it is better to let a fever run its course than to try to lower it. Let the fever run its course.

Flu symptoms usually last about 3 to 7 days. They often start improving gradually after the first 2 days. Keep in contact with your family doctor during this time should any additional symptoms occur.

## LACERATION (CUT)

Laceration can be taken care of in many different ways some don't even require stitches.

Each laceration will need to be assessed by a health care provider as to what treatment is needed.

Very large laceration or uncontrolled bleeding should be seen at a hospital contact emergency services.

Clean the laceration with clear water if possible. Apply pressure to stop any bleeding using a clean dressing. Ice will help reduce any swelling.

# LICE

Lice are tiny insect that live on clothing and your body. There are a few types of lice, head, body, and pubic area. It may take up to five days for the symptoms to disappear. Lice often recur.

Over the counter products work will to kill the lice and their eggs. A deep cleaning will be needed of your home, washing cloths, chairs, sofas etc. is the best way to reduce any re infestation.

Medical treatment by a health care provider is not needed. Diagnosis and self treatment can be done.

## MONONUCLEOSIS

Mono as most people know it is cause by a viral infection. Symptoms may include fever, sore throat, and fatigue.

It usually clears up in about 10 days but may take as long as 6 months. Tiredness can last for 2 to 6 weeks after other symptoms have cleared up.

# NOSEBLEEDS

Nose bleeds involves the blood vessels of one or both nostrils. Nose bleed can be caused by, injury, dry air, allergies or illnesses.

Most nose bleeds do not require medical attention. They can be controlled by applying direct pressure to nose and holding your head downward.

Direct pressure to the nose should be applied for at least 5 uninterrupted minutes. Don't swallow the blood this may upset your stomach. Refrain from blowing your nose.

## PNEUMONIA

Pneumonia can be cause by bacteria in the lungs. Symptoms may include, fever of 100.5 or more, cough, shortness of breath, chest pains, coughing up blood and fatigue. There are additional sign and systems. Chest X-rays and additional test maybe needed. Most pneumonia can be cured with antibiotics; some consumer may require hospitalization for I.V. antibiotics treatment.

# RASH

Rashes can result from infections, allergies, or irritation of the skin by chemicals or other environmental factors.

Rashes can also result from scratching or rubbing the skin too much to relieve itching.

Medical examination may be needed to identify the specific cause and proper treatment of your skin rash.

Notify your family doctor immediately If your rash is not better in 2-3 days. Signs of infection (increased pain, redness, drainage or pus). Or any fevers.

# SINUSITIS

Sinusitis is a condition consisting of inflammation of the sinuses, which may or may not be as a result of infection

Over the counter medication can relieve some of the symptoms. Which may include, headaches, face pressure, fatigue or pain.

Most of the time it will clear up on it own without antibiotics. If the symptoms last for more than 10 days antibiotic maybe needed.

## SORE THROATS

Inflammation of the throat in most cases it is painful and the initial infection can extend for a lengthy time. It can be accompanied by a cough or fever, if caused by an upper respiratory tract infection

Most cases are caused by viral infections (40%–60%),

Antibiotics don't work on viral infections, while bacterial causes may require antibiotics.

# SPRAINS

A sprain is an injury to ligaments that is caused by being stretched beyond their normal capacity. Pain, Swelling, Bruising Decreased ability to move the joint

The treatment of sprains depends on the extent of injury. Medications like non steroidal anti-inflammatory drugs can relieve pain.

Ice and compression will not completely stop swelling and pain, but will help to minimize them as the sprain begins to heal itself.

Careful management of swelling is critical to the healing process. Most minor sprain injuries recover without problems.

You may want to try the R.I.C.E. therapy as found near the end of this book.

# VOMITING

Causes of vomiting are sometimes is a viral infections. Vomiting can also be an important sign of other more serious illnesses. Dehydration is the other main concern with vomiting.

Giving small amounts of liquids should be give frequently to maintain hydration.

If vomiting last for more than two days or any blood contact your family doctor.

# WARTS

A wart is generally a small, rough tumor that can resemble a cauliflower or solid blister.

There are several over the counter options that should be tried first. Products are readily available at drugstores. There are typically two types of products: adhesive pad or a bottle removing a wart requires a strict regimen of cleaning, applying and removing the dead skin it may take up to 12 weeks to remove a wart.

Your family doctor or a dermatologist may have different treatment options if over the counter treatments have failed. Some can be painful, so be sure to discuss these risks with your health care provider.

## ADDITIONAL SERVICES

Expanding their reach deeper into the community, urgent aid clinics offer additional services to the local business. Some have added services to attract the business, such as workers compensation, pre employment physicals, physical therapy etc

Each area of country is different and each day new services are add but most included:

AED/CPR/First Aid Training
Hearing screenings
Health fairs
Drug testing
DOT Physicals
Immigration Physicals
Onsite workplace testing and training
Physical Therapy
Weight loss programs
Worker compensation evaluation
X-ray's

## DISCOUNTS

Urgent aid clinic have started a wave within their own waters. By offering the consumer discount coupons. Discount membership plans. Cash discounts are made for anyone who want to pay for services or for the under insured.

## MEDICATION FILLED ONSITE.

As an added benefit to Its customers, most urgent aid clinics will offer convenient onsite filling of your prescription. Some are able to bill your insurance directly for you. Most urgent aid clinic with ask for payment of your medication at the time of service. Some clinic may offer to submit your claim forms for you.

## MEDICAL EQUIPMENT

Urgent aid clinic offer medical supplies and equipment which include but not limited to crutches, ace wraps, cold pack etc.

Some insurance company may be billed while others require payment at the time of service.

## ONSITE TESTING

The most common onsite tests done at the urgent aid clinic are influenza, strep, mono, glucose, pregnancy, urinalysis, and ulcers can be done in about 20 minutes

## LAB TESTING

More advance testing will require lab testing few urgent aid clinics have onsite labs for these advance test.

You should ask for more information before you have these tests done. Most lab specimens will be sent to an outside lab.

There may be a time when the consumer may be asked to go directly to the lab or hospital for this advance test.

Most labs report result in about 72 hours after the specimen is received in the lab for testing.

# X-RAYS

Digital X-rays are the common norm today, very few clinic, hospitals, or doctors office use the old film technology anymore.

Some urgent aid clinics also provide x-ray services to other doctors offices. or clinics.

# MY MEDICAL HISTORY

This information is provided as a guild that will be helpful in writing your own medical history or for each of your family members. You can use a index card or a spiral notebook.

You should bring all this information with you when you or your family members seek **any** medical attention. Keep this information up to date. The following is a list of items that should be included in your medical history.

Birth date, detail of delivery and any complication that took place.

Serious and chronic illnesses and treatments.

Minor illnesses, infections or problems (ears infections etc.)

Drugs prescribed, (List names, amount, strength)

List nonprescription drugs or supplements.

Allergies to medication, foods, plants etc.

Immunizations include dates.

Medical test done and results.

Operations and hospitalizations
Include injuries and accidents or any time
loss of work due to medical problems.

Family history significant diseases of your
grandparents, parents, siblings etc.

Additional information you may include:

People to contact in an emergency
Doctors name, address and phone numbers.
Health insurance information.
Organ donor authorization.

# IMMUNIZATIONS

Vaccination should always be current for both adults and children. Keep a vaccination record for every member of your household.

Every health department, school, and medical clinic has a list of recommended vaccination with a schedule of when they should be given.

The most common vaccination are:

DTaP - protects against diphtheria, whooping cough (pertussis), and tetanus.

POLIO - protects against the virus that can cause paralysis and death.

MMR- Protect against measles, mumps, and rubella (German measles)

CHCKENPOX- protects against this mild disease.

HEPATITIS B - protects against a disease of the liver.

HIB – protects against Hemophilia influenza type B an infection of the brain, bones, throat and other areas.

PNEUMOCOCCAL CONJUGATE – protect against a diseases that can cause brain damage.

Many schools, colleges require proof of vaccinations.

# RICE THERAPY

R.I.C.E. is a acronym which stand for:

R-REST
I-ICE
C-COMPRESSION
E-ELEVATION

This can be used for any injury involving muscle or tendons.

Rest or stop using the injured part for a least 48 hours. Additional exercise could cause additional injury or delay healing.

Ice reduces swelling, ice the area for 20 minutes and least four times a day for the first 48 hours.

Compression decreases swelling by limiting the accumulation of blood near the injury site. Elastic bandage works very well. Do not wrap the area so tight that it impaired blood flow. Signs of poor blood flow numbness, cramping, or color changes in skin or nail beds.

If these symptoms appear remove the bandage. Rewrap only after symptoms have disappeared.

Elevation of the injury above the heart, too decrease swelling. Prop the arm or leg up with pillows.

If there is any increase pain, or swelling contact your family doctor.

## LIVING LONGER & HEALTHIER

Here are a few suggestions for healthier living. Some health problems can be reduced by factors we can all change.

Start by eating a healthier diet, limiting the amount of fats we eat. Try to eat one food for each food group during each and every meal.

Limiting snacks between meals. Can help you loose those unwanted pounds.

Where ever possible eat at the same times each day, don't skip meals. Avoid eating before you go to bed.

Exercise! Walk, run, dance, ride a bike or any physical activity it is that you enjoy.  Exercise for at least 20 to 30 minutes each and every day.

Don't smoke, smoking can reduce your life span.

Reduce the amount of alcohol you drink or don't drink at all. Beside the added health benefit think of the money you can save.

78

Avoid drugs and alcohol can impair your thinking process and lead to additional health problems.

Be involved to social activities, talk and visit friends and family regularly.

Get regular check up from both with your family doctor and dentist.

Get enough sleep, each and everyday. The bedroom should be used to relax, sleep and intimacy. Not as a place to catch up on work, or other stressful activities.

Use safety equipment whenever you can. Wear your seat belt when you ride in a car. Wear a helmet when you ride your bike.

The list of health tips can go on and on. We would like to hear your tips and ideas. My email address has been provided for you in the contacting us section of this book.

## CONTACTING US

No book can address every topic or every need of the vast amount of readers. We look forward to your suggestions, your stories of your experiences in our modern health care system.

For everyone that responds with a suggestion or comment you will receive a discount of 25% off the regular price of our next book.

## URGENT AID

## THE NEW HEALTHCARE CRISIS

I would like to take time to thank each reader for taking the time to learn more each and every day.

### *Thanks!*

NewFamilyDoctor@Aol.Com

###